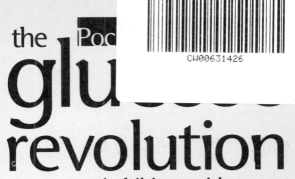

the Poc
glucose
revolution
and children with type 1
diabetes

ASSOC. PROFESSOR JENNIE BRAND-MILLER • KAYE FOSTER-POWELL
HEATHER GILBERTSON • DR ANTHONY LEEDS

coronet

First published in Australia in 2001 by
Hodder Headline Australia Pty Limited

First published in Great Britain in 2002 by Hodder and Stoughton
A division of Hodder Headline

This United Kingdom edition is published by arrangement with
Hodder Headline Australia Pty Limited
A Coronet paperback

10 9 8 7 6 5 4 3 2 1

A CIP catalogue record for this title is available from the British Library

0 340 77059 7

Typeset in Minion and Gill Sans by
Phoenix Typesetting, Ilkley, West Yorkshire

Printed and bound in Great Britain by Omnia Books Ltd, Glasgow

Hodder and Stoughton
A division of Hodder Headline
338 Euston Road
London NW1 3BH

CONTENTS

A word of advice

There are many factors that can affect your blood sugar levels. If you have diabetes and you are struggling to control your blood sugar levels it is important to seek medical help. How much exercise you do, your weight, stress levels, total dietary intake and need for medication may have to be reassessed.

HOW TO USE THIS BOOK

This book is a guide to the G.I. factor and children with type 1 diabetes. Many young people with diabetes, and their parents, find that despite doing everything they are told, blood sugar levels remain too high. We don't promise to be able to change this but we do believe an understanding of the G.I. of foods is an advantage to anyone with diabetes.

- We explain which types of carbohydrate are best and why (page 12).
- We show how to include more of the right sort of carbohydrate in your diet (page 19).
- We provide practical hints for meal preparation and tips to help make the G.I. factor work for you throughout the day.
- We supply low G.I. menus (pages 60–65).
- We include an A–Z listing of over 300 foods with their G.I. factor, carbohydrate and fat count (page 70).

This book contains the latest information about carbohydrate and the optimum diet for people with diabetes.

The G.I. factor is the glucose revolution – it gives the true story about carbohydrate and the blood sugar connection. For young people with diabetes this can mean a new lease of life.

Health authorities all over the world stress the importance of high carbohydrate diets for good health and diabetes management. The question now is what type of carbohydrate is best for people with diabetes? Research on the glycaemic index (what we call the G.I. factor) has led to a glucose revolution and shows that different carbohydrate foods have dramatically different effects on blood sugar levels.

Understanding the G.I. factor has made an enormous difference to the diet and lifestyle of everyone with diabetes. We now know:

- Many traditionally taboo foods don't have the unfavourable effects on blood sugar they were believed to have.
- Diets with a low G.I. factor improve blood sugar control in people with type 1 and type 2 diabetes.
- Many more foods make up a healthy diet for someone with diabetes than was once believed.

WHY WE WROTE THIS BOOK

In our first book, *The Glucose Revolution* (Hodder & Stoughton, 2000), we described how different types of carbohydrate work in different ways and we showed that the G.I. factor is:

■ a proven guide to the real effects of foods on blood sugar levels, and

■ an easy and effective way to eat a healthy diet and control fluctuations in blood sugar.

Carbohydrate foods that break down quickly during digestion have the highest G.I. factors. Their blood sugar response is fast and high. Carbohydrate foods that break down slowly, releasing glucose gradually into the bloodstream, have low G.I. factors.

The rate of carbohydrate digestion has important implications for everybody, but in this book we show how it can help young people with type 1 diabetes.

We believe that the G.I. factor of carbohydrate foods is vital information that will help with young people's day-to-day efforts at blood sugar control.

WHAT IS DIABETES?

Diabetes is a chronic condition in which there is too much sugar (glucose) in the blood. Normally, when a food containing carbohydrate is eaten, it is broken down into sugar and absorbed from the gut into the bloodstream. The sugar is then carried around in the blood to the body's muscles and cells, where it is used for energy.

Keeping blood sugar levels normal needs the right amount of a hormone called **insulin**. Insulin drives the sugar out of the blood and into the body's muscles, where it is used to provide energy for the body. If there is not enough insulin or if the insulin does not do its job properly, diabetes develops. There are two main types of diabetes.

In general, children and young adults develop diabetes because they no longer make enough insulin (type 1 diabetes). People over the age of about 40 usually develop diabetes because their insulin does not do its job properly (type 2 diabetes).

Type 1, or insulin-dependent diabetes mellitus is most commonly diagnosed during childhood. It is sometimes called 'juvenile diabetes'. In this type of diabetes, the pancreas does not produce enough insulin, and multiple insulin injections are needed every day to replace the insulin deficit. Since the amount of insulin injected is a prescribed dose, it is important to regulate the intake of carbohydrate to maintain balanced blood sugar levels.

Children and teenagers with type 1 diabetes will always have type 1 diabetes and will remain insulin dependent for the rest of their lives unless gene therapy or transplants come along sooner than we think.

Type 2, or non-insulin-dependent diabetes mellitus usually occurs in people over 40. People with type 2 diabetes can still make their own insulin, but their bodies are resistant to the actions of insulin. Exercise and taking care with what they eat is all that some people with type 2 diabetes have to do to keep their blood sugar levels within the normal range. Others also need to take tablets or insulin injections.

WHAT DOES THE GLUCOSE REVOLUTION MEAN FOR PEOPLE WITH DIABETES?

Not long ago, people with diabetes were told to eat complex carbohydrates (starches) because it was believed these were slowly absorbed, causing a smaller rise in blood sugar levels. Simple sugars were restricted because they were thought to be quickly absorbed and their blood sugar response would therefore be fast and high.

We now know that these assumptions were wrong. Different carbohydrate foods *do* have different effects on blood sugar levels, but we can't predict the effect by looking at the sugar or starch content. We know this because since the 1980s scientists have studied the actual blood sugar responses of healthy people and people with diabetes to hundreds of different foods. People were given real foods (i.e. not pure starches or pure sugars) and their blood sugar levels were then measured frequently for 2–3 hours after the meal.

To compare foods according to their true physiological effect on blood sugar levels, the scientists came up with the term 'glycaemic index' (what we call the G.I.). This is simply a ranking of foods from 0 to 100 that tells us whether a food will raise blood sugar levels dramatically, moderately or just a little (for more information see page 66).

The first surprise was that many starchy foods(bread,

potatoes, biscuits and many breakfast cereals) were digested and absorbed very quickly, not slowly as had always been assumed.

The next surprise was that moderate amounts of many sugary foods did not produce dramatic rises in blood sugar as had always been thought. Many foods containing sugar actually showed intermediate blood sugar responses, often lower than foods like bread.

The G.I. factor tells the true story. The old distinctions between starchy and sugary foods or simple versus complex carbohydrate have no scientific basis.

Think low G.I.

Forget about simple and complex carbohydrate.
Think glucose revolution!

WHY IS THE G.I. FACTOR SO IMPORTANT IN DIABETES?

If blood sugar levels are not properly controlled, diabetes can cause damage to the blood vessels in the heart, legs, brain, eyes and kidneys. This is why people with diabetes are at greater risk from heart attacks, strokes, kidney failure and blindness. High blood sugar levels can also damage the nerves in the feet, causing pain, irritation and numbness.

Low G.I. foods can help reduce the complications of diabetes by:

- improving blood sugar control, and
- improving blood fats.

Several studies show that a low G.I. diet lowers bad (LDL) cholesterol levels while increasing good (HDL) cholesterol. Increased levels of good HDL cholesterol are considered particularly protective against blood vessel disease and heart attack.

*The slow digestion and gradual rise and fall
in blood sugar after a low G.I. food
help control blood sugar levels for people
with diabetes.*

HOW FOOD AFFECTS BLOOD SUGAR

Our bodies burn fuel all the time and the fuel our bodies like best is carbohydrate. In fact, carbohydrate is the *only* fuel that our brains and red blood cells can use. This includes starchy foods such as bread, potatoes, pasta, rice and noodles plus natural sugar foods, like fruit and milk, and all the added sugar foods like ice-cream, jam, chocolate, soft drink and lollies.

Digestion starts in the mouth as we chew our food, and amylase, the digestive enzyme in saliva, is incorporated into the food. The digestive action of this enzyme stops in the stomach. Most digestion after this takes place in the small intestine where amylase from pancreatic juice breaks down the large molecules of starch into short-chain molecules. These and any disaccharide sugars are then broken into simpler monosaccharides by enzymes in the wall of the intestine. The monosaccharides that result (glucose, fructose and galactose) are absorbed from the small intestine into the bloodstream.

Our bodies respond by releasing insulin into the bloodstream. This clears the sugar from the blood with some moving into the muscles and cells where it is used for energy and some being stored in the liver for use later on. Some glucose is maintained in the blood to serve the brain and central nervous system.

WHAT'S GOOD FOR PEOPLE WITH DIABETES IS GOOD FOR EVERYBODY

With insulin injections, blood tests, time schedules and the need to eat regularly, the pursuit of normal blood sugar levels can seem endless. While we don't claim to have all the answers we do know that the G.I. factor can help you – whether it improves your blood sugar levels or just explains why some foods have the effects you've observed. A diet that is good for people with diabetes is a diet that is good for everybody, because it is a healthy, balanced diet that contains a wide variety of foods.

When you are deciding what to eat, taste is very important. But it is also worth giving some thought to:

- how hungry you are
- how the food may affect your blood sugar
- what nutrients your body needs
- the variety of foods you eat throughout the day, and
- what activity you're doing.

FOR PARENTS

The body has different nutritional requirements at different ages, and this is taken into account when planning the diet for a child with diabetes. As your child grows, you will need to review and adjust his or her diet with the help of a dietitian.

HOW DOES INSULIN WORK?

Our bodies normally make insulin so that we can use carbohydrate for energy. Insulin works like a key to unlock the cells and let the sugar move out of the blood and into them. The body usually makes just enough insulin to keep blood sugars at the right level.

However, if you have type 1 diabetes you have to rely on insulin injections to do this. Usually the insulin dose is pretty much the same from day to day, and you plan a regular carbohydrate intake to balance the insulin dose. All this sounds simple in theory, but in practice it can be hard to keep blood sugars at the right level. One reason is that many other things besides food affect your blood sugar levels – such as the activity you are doing, how long it's been since you last ate, and what your other hormones are up to.

Another reason why it can be hard to keep blood sugars at the right level is that when it comes to food, your blood sugar is affected not only by how much carbohydrate you eat but also by the type of carbohydrate you eat.

WHAT TYPE OF CARBOHYDRATE?

Thanks to research on the G.I. factor we now know that foods containing sugar can be enjoyed in moderation as a normal part of a healthy diet for someone with diabetes. Sugar itself has only an intermediate G.I. value, which means it has a moderate effect on blood sugar levels compared with other carbohydrate foods. Many foods containing sugar, such as yoghurt and flavoured milk, actually have low G.I. factors and raise blood sugar levels less than regular bread.

Many of you will be familiar with the carbohydrate exchange system that has been used for many years to give people with diabetes guidance on how much carbohydrate to eat. The G.I. research, however, has scientifically proven that this system is flawed. The exchange system assumes that equal amounts of different carbohydrate foods have similar effects on blood sugar levels. This is incorrect. The change in your blood sugar after one exchange of cornflakes, for example, is very different from that after one exchange of apple.

While you may find the carbohydrate exchange system is a helpful guide to carbohydrate quantity, remember its limitations when it comes to predicting the impact of foods on your blood sugar levels.

4 tips for choosing carbohydrate

- ■ Use standard household measures so that the amount of carbohydrate consumed remains consistent.
- ■ Eat regular meals and snacks based on carbohydrate foods.
- ■ Choose your carbohydrate from a wide variety of sources – both starch and sugar foods.
- ■ Use the G.I. tables to choose the most suitable carbohydrate for you.

FOR PARENTS

What's a serving?

A carbohydrate serving is simply a way of ensuring that there is daily consistency in the amount of carbohydrate eaten at various meals. Many diabetes clinics work on a set carbohydrate serving which roughly corresponds to the size of a slice of bread, a medium size piece of fruit or simply the amount that fits in the palm of the child's hand. It is important with serving sizes to be consistent from one day to the next.

Be aware

Products labelled 'low calorie' contain little or no carbohydrate and will not affect blood sugar levels. However excessive use of artificially sweetened products is neither recommended nor necessary in a well-balanced, low G.I. diet.

A WORD ABOUT FAT

Although fat doesn't directly affect blood sugar levels, it certainly can't be ignored. The fat we eat affects our body weight, cholesterol levels, risk of diabetic complications and chance of poor health from everyday diseases like obesity, heart disease and even cancer.

A low fat diet is *not recommended* for very young children, but it's fine for children over five years of age to eat low fat products. Keep in mind that the omega-3 fats found in fish are important sources of 'good' fat to eat regularly.

If you need to control weight, limiting total fat intake is important and you should consult a dietitian. Otherwise, just think about the type of fat you eat. Polyunsaturated fats, found in some margarines and vegetable oils, and monounsaturated fats, such as olive oil, blended vegetable oils and rapeseed oil, are preferable to saturated fats, such as butter and fatty meats. Limiting saturated fats is recommended for everyone. It's particularly important for children because the changes in blood vessels that lead to heart disease begin in childhood. Check out the list of sources of saturated fats on page 15, and you'll see that limiting saturated fats requires diligence!

HIGH FAT FOODS TO WATCH OUT FOR

Butter

Cakes, biscuits

Cheese

Chicken nuggets

Chips – hot, fried

Coconut milk and cream

Corn chips

Cream

Doughnuts

Fat – solid cooking fats and cooking margarines; white fat on beef, lamb, pork

French fries

Ice-creams

Pastries

Pies

Pizza with meat and cheese toppings

Potato crisps

Sausages

Takeaways – most Asian takeaways and most fast foods

Thickshakes and milkshakes

GETTING FOOD RIGHT THROUGH EXERCISE

Good health, a reasonable body weight and good blood sugar levels are all easier to achieve if you exercise, because your insulin will work better.

*Exercise means being active every day –
whether playing sport, taking part in an active
hobby or walking the dog around the block.*

Activity outside your normal routine may mean you need to eat extra carbohydrate. This is just a precaution to prevent your blood sugar levels dropping too low. Just how much extra you need will depend on your level of fitness, the type of activity and the amount of effort. As a rough guide, one extra serving of carbohydrate is suggested for every hour of strenuous activity. Generally, the more strenuous and the longer the duration of the exercise, the more additional carbohydrate is required.

Your usual insulin dose and food intake covers normal play activities – even quite strenuous ones.

SUSTAINING YOUR BLOOD SUGAR LEVELS DURING EXERCISE

■ If you are eating immediately before exercising, select foods with a high G.I. – sweet biscuits, sweets, muesli bars, cordial or a normal bread sandwich.

■ If you are eating 1–2 hours before exercising, choose foods with a low G.I. – yoghurt, a sandwich made from low G.I. bread, low G.I. cereals, low G.I. fruits, milkshakes or 2-minute noodles.

■ If you need to eat during prolonged exercise (over an hour) choose foods with a high G.I. that you can 'eat on the run'. Sports drinks and cordials may be best as they meet both fuel and fluid requirements.

■ If you are eating between events throughout the day (e.g. school sports days, bike races, a day at the beach) choose a combination of low and high G.I. foods. It is generally appropriate to decrease the usual insulin dose by 10 per cent as well so that an excessive intake of food is not necessary.

■ If additional foods are required to restore blood sugar levels after exercise, choose foods with a high G.I. – rice crackers, white bread, watermelon or a high G.I. cereal. Drink plenty of water, too, or select high G.I. drinks to meet carbohydrate and fluid needs simultaneously.

SOME BLOOD SUGAR GUIDELINES
Your blood sugar will tend to fall during exercise

If it is less than 10 mmol/L before exercise, you may need extra carbohydrate before, during and after exercise to prevent hypoglycaemia. If it is more than 15 mmol/L and ketones are present in your urine before exercise, postpone exercise until overall control has improved. Otherwise, exercise may actually increase your blood sugar levels further.

(Ketones are a product of fat breakdown that occurs when insufficient insulin is available. Without adequate insulin, the body is unable to utilise its preferred fuel, glucose, so it uses fat instead. The concentration of sugar in the blood is measured as the concentration of sugar molecules (moles) per litre. One thousand millimoles (mmol) equals one mole and one mole of glucose is 180 grammes.)

EVERYONE RESPONDS TO EXERCISE DIFFERENTLY

Because of this you may need extra carbohydrate before and/or doing and/or after exercise, and the quantity you need may also vary. You will learn from experience what suits you best. Initially, monitoring blood sugar before, during and after exercise will give you the best indication of how your body responds.

CARBOHYDRATE FOODS AND LOW G.I. CHOICES

For a low G.I. diet include at least one low G.I. carbohydrate per meal.

Breads – Fruit Loaf and Mixed Grain breads; Multigrain breads; Stoneground Wholemeal

Breakfast Cereals – All-Bran™ Original, Fruit 'n' Oats, Frosties™, Special K™, Mini-Wheats™, natural muesli, porridge, semolina

Fresh fruits – apples, apricots, bananas, cherries, custard apple, grapes, kiwi-fruit, mango, oranges, paw paw, peaches, pears, plums

Dried fruits – apples, apricots, sultanas

Grains – barley, pasta, noodles, sweet corn, buckwheat, Basmati rice, couscous

Vegetables – baked beans, butter (cannellini) beans, kidney beans, lentils, chickpeas, sweet corn, lima beans, sweet potato

Dairy foods – milk, yoghurt, ice-cream, custard, flavoured milk, mousse

HANDLING HYPOS

Hypoglycaemia (hypo) means a low level of sugar in the blood, usually below 3.0–4.0 mmol/L. It may be caused by:

- taking too much insulin
- vigorous exercise without extra carbohydrate
- missing or delaying meals, or
- not eating an adequate amount of carbohydrate food.

The way you feel when your blood sugar is low varies from person to person. Common symptoms are excessive sweating, tiredness, drowsinesss, irritability, dizziness, shaking, headache and blurred vision.

Learn the signs of a hypo and act quickly.
If hypos happen often, contact your doctor or
diabetes nurse specialist so your insulin dose can
be reviewed.

WHAT TO DO ABOUT HYPOS

- Consume some quickly absorbed (high G.I.) carbohydrate (jellybeans, soft drink, Lucozade™). This will immediately increase the blood sugar levels. Repeat again in 5 minutes if there is no improvement.
- Soon after (10–15 minutes), follow with an intermediate or low G.I. carbohydrate food (bread, biscuits, fruit, milk). This will prevent the hypo recurring.
- Always carry foods to treat hypos.
- The extra foods you eat because you have a hypo are *extra* and should not be subtracted from your next meal or snack.
- Do not leave someone who has had a hypo unattended until they are feeling better.
- Try to work out why the hypo occurred so as to prevent it happening again. Most hypos are preventable but some occur for no apparent reason.

FOR PARENTS

A word about toddler tantrums

Tantrums are common with independent toddlers. Sometimes it's difficult to determine whether a toddler is irritable due to hypoglycaemia or just having a typical 'terrible twos' tantrum. When in doubt, remember it is potentially more dangerous to **not** treat the hypoglycaemia in a young child.

COPING WITH NIGHT-TIME HYPOS

Hypoglycaemia can occur at night. Most of the time, children wake when they are experiencing a hypo, or at least they become very restless so that their parents wake. Sometimes, however, children sleep soundly through a hypo and the body self-corrects and overcompensates, which shows up as high blood sugar readings the next morning.

Minimising the risk of night-time hypoglycaemia

■ Eat a supper that emphasises food with a low G.I. factor (see snack suggestions on page 58).

■ Test blood sugars before bed, after checking with your doctor about what is an appropriate pre-bed level. You may need some extra carbohydrate.

■ Don't skip supper, even if the evening blood sugar test is high. Eating a low G.I. food for supper is the best choice.

FOR PARENTS

Occasionally check your child's blood sugar readings at 2.00 a.m. This is important if you suspect night-time hypoglycaemia or if your child is unwell, has eaten poorly over the day or has had unusually high activity levels.

WHAT TO DO WHEN YOUR CHILD IS SICK

Your child is likely to get coughs and colds and all the normal childhood illnesses. Unfortunately, these can make diabetes hard to manage. Loss of appetite is partly the cause. It is essential to monitor blood sugars closely during an illness.

- **Always give insulin**. The liver is still producing (perhaps overproducing) glucose to maintain blood sugar levels. Insulin is essential in order to manage this output.
- Monitor blood sugar levels very closely (every 2 hours).
- Test all urine for ketones. The presence of ketones requires immediate attention and extra insulin will be needed.
- Continue to give carbohydrate in some form and ensure an adequate fluid intake.

If ever in doubt when managing a child with diabetes who is sick, do not hesitate to contact your diabetes doctor or diabetes nurse specialist for additional advice.

SICK DAY BLOOD SUGARS

If blood sugar readings are greater than 12 mmol/L

Give low calorie fluids (water, diet drinks). You may give slightly fewer carbohydrate foods while the sugar remains high since you are monitoring the readings more frequently. Don't omit carbohydrate foods.

If blood sugar readings are less than 12 mmol/L

Give carbohydrate in some form. Choosing foods from the intermediate G.I. range will help sustain blood sugar levels while food intake is reduced. Try:

plain toast	ice-cream	stewed fruit
dry biscuits	milkshakes	fruit juices
sweet biscuits	soup	potato crisps

If your child's appetite is poor, use intermediate to high G.I. foods eaten or sipped frequently. It is often easier for your child to have a little and often. Try offering:

sweetened soft drink	sweetened jelly	jellybeans
Lucozade™	icy poles	lollipops

If your child has diarrhoea, sweet fluids *must* be diluted with water (one part water, one part soft drink). Avoid giving full-strength sweet fluid, as it may actually worsen the diarrhoea.

BABIES WITH DIABETES

Breastfeeding is best for babies with diabetes. Let your baby dictate how much, but monitor blood sugars routinely. If breastfeeding is not possible, offer an infant formula at least every 3–4 hours.

Breast milk or infant formula should be your baby's main drink up to 12 months of age. When your baby is about 7 months, you can introduce full-cream cows' milk in small quantities as custard, yoghurt or on cereal. From 12 months, when your baby is eating a varied diet, you can offer full-cream cows' milk as the main drink.

Encourage dairy foods because not only are they an important source of calcium but they have low G.I. values – a big advantage when trying to optimise your baby's blood sugar control.

You can begin introducing solids (including low G.I. ones) from 4–6 months when your baby is ready. By 12 months your baby should be enjoying the family meal with you and drinking full-cream cows' milk from a cup. Serve the whole family delicious low G.I. meals. Our books *The Glucose Revolution* and *G.I. Plus* contain hundreds of recipes, and meal and snack ideas for everybody.

RECOMMENDED DAILY QUANTITIES OF FOOD IN BABY'S FIRST YEAR

Age in months	Food	Texture	Suggested daily amount
4–6	Iron-fortified rice cereal	Pureed/strained	1–3 tablespoons
	Soft cooked vegetables and fruit (be sure to include low G.I. varieties)		1–3 tablespoons
	Breast milk or infant formula		On demand 180–240 mL x 4 feeds/day
6–8	Soft cooked vegetables Stewed, tinned or soft ripe fruit (encourage low G.I. varieties)	Pureed/mashed	2–4 tablespoons
	Iron-fortified rice cereal and other cereals (select low G.I. cereals where appropriate)		2–4 tablespoons
	Pureed meat, chicken and fish. Start to offer egg yolk		1–2 tablespoons
	Breast milk or infant formula		On demand 240 mL x 3–4 feeds/day

Age in months	Food	Texture	Suggested daily amount
8–10	Cereals: rice cereals, wheatflake biscuits, porridge Multigrain bread/toast, fruit loaf (encourage low G.I. varieties)	Pureed/mashed Offer finger foods (chopped pieces)	2–5 tablespoons
	Mashed fruits and vegetables (encourage low G.I. varieties)		3–5 tablespoons
	Minced meats, flaked fish, whole egg, cheese sticks		3–5 tablespoons
	Breast milk or infant formula		On demand 240 mL x 3 feeds/day from bottle or cup
10–12	Wide variety from five food groups: cereals and breads, fruit and vegetables, dairy products, meat and meat alternatives, fats and oils (select low G.I. varieties where appropriate)	Chopped	According to child's appetite
	Breast milk or infant formula		On demand 240 mL x 3 feeds/day from bottle or cup

DEAR HEATHER

How can I tell if my breastfed baby is getting enough breast milk to avoid hypoglycaemia?

If your baby is thriving, has several wet nappies a day, appears settled after feeds and is demand feeding 2–3 hourly over the day, the chances are that your baby is receiving enough and doing well. Regular monitoring of his blood sugar levels will also reassure you that his needs are being met.

Should I introduce solids earlier?

No. There is no benefit in introducing solids before 4–6 months of age. A baby's digestive system is still immature and not ready to cope with solid foods before 4 months. Introducing foods earlier may increase your baby's chances of developing food allergies, diarrhoea (due to undigested food) and poor growth. If you think your baby is hungry, offer more breast milk or formula feeds until she is ready to start solids.

What is the best way to manage a hypo for an infant?

When hypoglycaemia occurs, treat by giving glucose syrup either on a dummy or a soft plastic spoon, followed by a breast or formula feed.

TODDLERS AND PRESCHOOLERS WITH DIABETES

Although toddlers like to explore and show their independence, they are still too young to understand their specific dietary needs. This can sometimes cause difficulties when they are with friends, at playgroup or when grown-ups 'spoil' them with an excess of treats. Picky eating and food fads are also common.

Toddlers don't eat as much simply because they don't need as much. Refusing food is also a way for them to express their newfound independence. Don't fuss or pay special attention, as a hungry toddler will never starve.

However, when you add diabetes to the equation, and hence the need for regular carbohydrate to prevent hypoglycaemia, you can understand why parents become anxious. But bribing, bullying and fussing usually only make matters worse.

The best way to cope with food refusal is to try to avoid the whole situation. Allow your toddler to graze throughout the day according to appetite rather than expecting him to eat set meals at set times. Use these strategies to try to defuse the situation:

- ■ **Don't panic**. Don't resort to circus tricks as this gives him the impression that refusing food gains lots of attention.
- ■ **Bargain calmly**. Try to get the carbohydrate foods in first; for example, 'You can leave your egg if you eat your toast.'
- ■ **Try substituting**. Substitute the refused food with another healthy food that you know your toddler likes. Offer only one alternative each time or this can become a game of choices. Don't offer indulgent snack foods as an alternative.
- ■ **Try finger foods and snacks**. If your toddler still refuses to eat, leave finger foods (fruit pieces, savoury biscuits or sandwich fingers) nearby so he can nibble as he plays.
- ■ **Try distraction**. Sitting your toddler on your lap and reading a book can be a good distraction and may encourage eating.
- ■ **Be prepared for a hypo**. When all else fails be prepared for a hypo. Use Lucozade™ or soft drink. Do not treat the hypo with jellybeans or lollies as he may regard this as a reward for not eating his meal and hence reinforce the food refusal behaviour.

IF FOOD REFUSAL CONTINUES TO BE AN ISSUE

Reducing the insulin dose temporarily may be warranted to minimise the risk of hypoglycaemia and to reduce tension and anxiety until food intake improves.

Remember, there's no single food that your toddler must eat. Encourage him to enjoy exploring new tastes and sensations in unchallenged and comfortable surroundings.

Introduce new foods together with familiar foods that your toddler likes. Try offering them at several different meals and with other children who like to eat those foods. Never force him to eat, as this may encourage food refusal behaviours. Respect your toddler's wishes if he says he is full. Encourage him during the mealtime so he feels confident about trying new tastes – and thinks mealtime's fun.

RECOMMENDED DAILY QUANTITIES OF FOOD FOR TODDLERS AND PRESCHOOLERS

Food group	Suggested daily amount
Bread and cereals (encourage wholegrain breads, low G.I. cereals, pasta, low G.I. rice)	4–5 servings
Fruit and vegetables (encourage low G.I. varieties)	3–4 servings
Meat and meat alternatives (include low G.I. legumes and pulses)	1–2 servings (30–60 g)
Milk and dairy (all varieties are low G.I. sources)	3 servings (600 ml)
Margarine and oils	2–3 teaspoons (10 g)

Try to include a minimum of one low G.I. food per meal per day to achieve good long-term diabetes control.

DEAR HEATHER

My toddler is so tired by the end of the day, he won't eat his evening meal and I am frightened that he will hypo in the middle of the night. What should I do?

It is not unusual for tired toddlers not to want dinner. Feeding a toddler with diabetes earlier (5.00–5.30 p.m.) may help; then he can eat with the family later without the pressure of having to have a certain amount of food. Any extra carbohydrate foods then will be a bonus.

Alternatively, try giving toddlers their main meal at midday, when their appetite is better. This means you can offer a lighter evening meal – sandwiches, fruit or yoghurt.

Make sure your toddler has at least one low G.I. food in his evening meal or supper snack. Check the meal and snack suggestions (page 58–65) for ways to incorporate low G.I. foods into his usual food choices. A bottle or cup of milk has a low G.I. and is a common bedtime routine. Add honey to boost carbohydrate intake if necessary.

The occasional night-time blood sugar test before you go to bed may also be reassuring.

My two-year-old girl's blood sugars are never stable.
How can I work out what I am doing wrong?

Be reassured that you are not the only parent of a
toddler with diabetes who is frustrated with unstable
diabetes control. We do not aim for tight control
because of the difficulties in detecting and treating
hypos. Toddlers are too young to recognise hypo
symptoms. A wider blood sugar range is acceptable
in this age group because their activity levels are
erratic and their food intake can be unpredictable.
The HbA1c result from clinic is often a better indication of their overall diabetes control than the
highly fluctuating daily blood tests. (The level of
HbA1c is a measure of the *average* level of blood
sugars over the previous 6–8 weeks.)

Incorporating low G.I. foods over the course of the
day may help by minimising the rapid fluctuations in
blood sugars that are often observed, but it certainly
won't prevent them. If you can manage your
toddler's diabetes so that she is hypo free and ketone
free, you are doing a *fabulous* job.

My two-year-old son is about to start childcare. How can I be sure that his diabetes will be managed properly?

One of the hardest things about being parent is letting go as your toddler becomes more independent and others assume responsibility. You need to feel confident that the staff are able to manage his diabetes. They need to be made aware of his usual routines and also how to recognise and treat symptoms of hypoglycaemia.

In our experience, there have been no difficulties with children attending childcare. The days are structured to a routine and the meals supplied are nutritious and appropriate. The diabetes nurse specialist at your clinic may be able to visit the centre or provide you with written information to pass on to the staff.

THE PRIMARY SCHOOL CHILD WITH DIABETES

Once at school, children with diabetes usually become more independent and start to take on aspects of their own diabetes care. This should be encouraged, although parents need to continue supporting and supervising. The majority of children in this age group are on two injections per day, pre-breakfast and pre-dinner. Blood testing during the school day is usually not required, so children with diabetes can attend school without having to deal with the hassles of injections and finger pricks.

The lunch box look!

At school, lunch boxes are compared, and swaps and trade-offs begin. It is important that your child has an understanding of her diet and carbohydrate foods so she can make appropriate lunch swaps. You can do this by involving her when you are preparing the school lunch. Pack enough foods to cover break-time and lunch, and possibly extra for sports or after-school activities. Try to include an interesting selection of low G.I. food choices for each day and vary the contents regularly so she doesn't become bored. It's very important for children with diabetes that the contents of their lunch boxes don't look too different from what their friends are eating. Provide a nutritious, wholesome lunch box by basing the contents on the combinations given on page 58.

- Don't worry if your child selects the same foods for her lunch box every day as long as her food choices are mainly healthy. She will let you know when she's bored and ready for variation.
- Make sure an adequate amount of carbohydrate food is packed each day to meet your child's needs for lunch, snacks, sports and unexpected extras.

What to do about a late-morning break

A common problem for many school children is a delayed morning break-time, because break is usually around 11.00 a.m. at school. Often this gap between breakfast and morning break is too long and hypoglycaemia may occur.

Some children try to eat during class to prevent the hypo but this singles them out and may make them feel uncomfortable. Others have a small low G.I. snack – dried apricots, flavoured milk, a small yoghurt, or dry biscuits with cheese spread – either on the way to school or before first bell to hold the blood sugar steady. This way they can have morning tea with the other children at break and not have to worry about a hypo.

No need to be a party pooper!

Your child should not miss out on party fun and fare just because she has diabetes. Within reason, relax her diet for that special meal or snack. Allow a moderate number of party treats. Having one slice of birthday cake is sensible, but going back for a third helping is not. Encourage her to bring home the lollies which can either be dessert that evening or eaten prior to exercise later. An occasional rise in blood sugar levels on special occasions does no harm. It's what you do the remainder of the time that is important.

On the day of the party, keep the insulin dose the same (even though it is likely that she'll eat extra). Remember she may be more active at the party, which would allow her to eat the extra party food without increasing blood sugar levels too dramatically.

If blood sugars are high after the party, don't panic. Make sure she eats her dinner and supper so her blood sugar levels don't drop rapidly overnight.

Many parents are surprised at how good their child's blood sugar readings are after parties.

Hypoglycaemia at school

Hypoglycaemia can occur at school, so make sure your child is prepared. Organising a 'hypo box' for school is a good idea. It should include favourite high G.I. plus some low G.I. non-perishable finger foods – jellybeans, soft lollies, fruit drinks, Lucozade™, portion-pack dry biscuits, muesli bars, etc.

It's a good idea to leave a couple of hypo boxes in strategic locations (one in the classroom, another in the sick bay or staffroom) along with a card describing clearly the appropriate treatment for your child's hypo. Replenish supplies regularly and check that foods are within their 'use-by' date.

If your child appears to have hypos at school more often than at home, you have to consider the possibility that he is 'faking' hypos to get sweets. One way you can address this problem is to do some blood testing at school to confirm whether hypoglycaemia is actually occurring. If it is, you will have to look for the reason and deal with it.

RECOMMENDED DAILY QUANTITIES OF FOOD FOR THE PRIMARY SCHOOL CHILD

Food group	Suggested daily amount
Bread and cereals (encourage wholegrain breads, low G.I. cereals, pasta, low G.I. rice)	4 or more servings
Fruit and vegetables (encourage low G.I. varieties)	5 or more servings
Meat and meat alternatives (include low G.I. legumes and pulses)	1 serving (100 g)
Milk and dairy (all varieties are low G.I. sources)	3 servings (600–800 ml)
Margarine and oils	3–4 teaspoons (15–20 g)

Try to include a minimum of one low G.I. food per meal per day to achieve good long-term diabetes control.

DEAR HEATHER

My daughter refuses to eat breakfast before going to school and I'm worried that she will hypo on the way to school. What should I do?

Skipping breakfast is not an option for any child with diabetes. Breakfast is an important meal to start the day. It is also a great opportunity to include plenty of low G.I. foods because many breads, cereals, fresh fruits and dairy foods have a low G.I. Some children do not have large appetites at breakfast time, so it is important to optimise carbohydrate intake.

Make sure there is plenty of time to enjoy a good breakfast. Milkshakes, fruit smoothies and hot chocolate drinks are good starters, with low G.I.s that will sustain blood sugar levels for longer periods. Negotiate foods that she will eat – they needn't necessarily be traditional breakfast foods. Check the low G.I. breakfast list (pages 60–61 for ideas).

She may prefer two small low G.I. snacks (one at breakfast and one on the way to school). This will ensure sufficient carbohydrate intake to minimise the risk of a hypo.

I spend weekends baking special sugar-free cakes and biscuits for my son's school lunch to try to give him more variety but these always come home uneaten. Can you suggest any special recipe books?

There is no need to use special sugar-free recipes or artificial sweeteners. Using moderate amounts of sugar in cooking is acceptable and will do no harm to diabetes control as part of total carbohydrate. Bake your family's favourite recipes, and remember that recipes are more likely to need their fat content modified than their sugar content.

When my son is invited to parties he gets so busy playing he hardly eats and always ends up hypo. What should I do?

Give your son a low G.I. snack before he goes to the party so it's not so important he eats there. It will help sustain his blood sugars and modify the effect on his blood sugar level of any party foods he does eat.

My child is very active during playtime at school so I pack a lolly in his lunch box every day to prevent a hypo. He eats more lollies now than he ever did before he was diagnosed with diabetes. Does this seem right?

Your child should **not** need lollies every day to prevent hypos. Even if he is very active at play, his regular insulin dose and food intake should be appropriate for his usual level of activity. Additional carbohydrate foods are only required for **extra strenuous** activity. If you find that your child needs extra foods regularly, review his insulin dose and/or offer other carbohydrate food choices.

JUST FOR TEENAGERS

Teenage years tend to be a time to challenge the world. And that includes smoking, drinking, skipping insulin, missing meals, eating whatever! In this section we provide information that will help you to make decisions in the interests of your long-term diabetes control and your day-to-day health.

Hollow legs?

Teenagers grow fast and get very hungry? Be flexible with your diet.

- When you are hungry, try low G.I. foods for maximum fill-up value – wholegrain bread, bananas, yoghurt, pasta.
- When you aren't so interested in eating, have high G.I. foods in smaller amounts – regular bread, biscuits, cornflakes.

Takeway food

The problem with takeaway foods is that they usually involve eating at irregular times and eating greater quantities of sugary and/or fatty foods than is recommended as part of a well-balanced low G.I. diet. Eating additional carbohydrate food will result in increased blood sugar levels.

But, you don't have to be different. Incorporating low

G.I. foods where practicable will let you enjoy takeaway foods without compromising diabetes control. Low G.I. foods include milkshakes, ice-creams, yoghurts, dried noodle snacks, popcorn and fresh fruit. Some other tips:

- Choose bottled water, flavoured milk or diet soft drinks in preference to regular soft drinks.
- When eating foods that contain high G.I. carbohydrates or saturated fats, combine them with other low G.I. foods.
- Be prepared. Have only a light snack after school so you have to have an extra snack with your friends.
- Organise your get-togethers before you play sport so the extra carbohydrate you have while socialising is burned up during the exercise.
- Walk or cycle home after socialising.

TAKEAWAY OPTIONS

Takeaway food	Best choices	Foods to limit
Fish and chips	Grilled fish Steamed dim sum	Deep fried varieties Chips
McDonald's, Burger King, etc.	Burgers with salad Diet drinks Mineral water Plain ice-cream sundae	Thickshakes Sweetened soft drinks
Hot chips	Potato wedges Baked potato with cheese and salad	
Pizza	Vegetarian pizza	Salami, double cheese topping
Burgers	Burger with meat and salad only	Double meat, extra cheese, fried onions, bacon
Chinese, Thai or Vietnamese	Stir-fried meat or chicken with steamed rice Stir fried veggies or noodles	Fried rice Deep fried spring rolls or dim sum Battered foods
Café or sandwich shop	Wholegrain roll or sandwich Milkshakes Frozen yoghurt	Pies, pasties, sausage rolls, battered savs, potato chips

Drinking alcohol and staying out late

Having diabetes doesn't mean you can't stay out late, sleep in and drink alcohol, but planning beforehand helps. Ask your doctor, diabetes nurse specialist or dietitian for advice. They can help because they have been through this before.

How does alcohol affect blood sugar levels?

Some drinks, like beer, sweet mixers, coolers and liqueurs, may initially cause hyperglycaemia (high blood sugars), but the biggest problem of combining alcohol with diabetes is hypoglycaemia because alcohol prevents the release of stored sugar from the liver. (Your body normally calls on these stores if your blood sugar levels drop too low.) Hypoglycaemia can go undetected if you've had too much to drink – the signs of a hypo and of being drunk are similar. Make sure that someone in your group knows that alcohol can make you hypo so that he or she can help you treat it if necessary.

Remember:
- Always carry extra food wherever you are going.
- Wear some form of diabetes ID (such as an ID bracelet) just in case.

Try low-alcohol beers, diluting wines with soda water and making long drinks with spirits and diet mixers. Diet Coke neat is also popular.

> *Guidelines on alcohol consumption in the UK and elsewhere indicate that intakes of more than two units* per day for women and three for men (whether with or without diabetes) are associated with high risk of alcohol-related disease.*

What to do with your insulin

Drinking on an empty stomach leads to higher blood alcohol levels and a greater risk of hypoglycaemia. Before you go out for the night, inject your insulin and eat a low G.I. meal – pasta is perfect. You may need to reduce your insulin dose and the timing of your doses if you've lined up lots of activity.

If you're on a twice daily insulin regimen, your usual routine need not be altered (apart from the need to snack regularly throughout the evening).

If you're on a basal bolus regimen (four injections per day given before each main meal and at suppertime), you can:

■ have your long-acting insulin with your short-acting pre-dinner injection and eat while out, or

* One unit = a glass of wine, ½ glass of beer, single measure of spirits.

■ have your long-acting insulin when you get home and eat a carbohydrate snack before going to bed.

Taking your long-acting insulin later means you can sleep in a little longer next morning. But, if you're taking your long-acting insulin very late, consider reducing the dose.

During the evening, snack regularly (at least two-hourly) on carbohydrate foods.

Test your blood sugar levels before going to bed. If you're hypo treat it, if not, have a quick snack. Something with a low G.I. would be good (wholegrain toast or a chocolate drink). This will minimise the risk of a hypo while you're asleep and will give you the extra carbohydrate you need to compensate for that inevitable sleep-in.

If you take your long-acting insulin injection later the previous night you can delay the following morning's injection to 10.00 a.m. – no later! Alternatively, take your morning insulin at the usual time (or no more than one hour later than usual), eat a light breakfast and go back to bed.

Delaying insulin injections for longer periods is not recommended because the action of different insulin types will overlap and make diabetes control unpredictable.

Weighty matters

Sometimes the pressures of having the body beautiful seem to clash with the diabetes-linked need to eat regularly, eat after exercise and treat hypos. But you can maintain a reasonable body weight and still look after your diabetes.

Becoming overweight is largely an imbalance between activity levels and food intake. If you honestly think you have a weight problem and you are worried about how you look and want to diet, talk to someone about it; ideally someone independent, like your doctor, diabetes nurse specialist or dietitian. They can provide you with some good options.

Carbohydrates are natural appetite suppressants. And of all carbohydrate foods, those with a low G.I. factor are among the most filling and prevent hunger pangs for longer.

Here's a list of don'ts because they *don't* work!

- Don't eliminate a major food group like meat or dairy foods in the belief they are fattening foods. The result is a nutritionally inadequate intake with detrimental long-term consequences.

- Don't try a severe low calorie diet either, because it can dramatically affect your growth and development – and that includes your brain. It's also counter-productive to long-term weight control.

- Don't reduce, or worse still, skip insulin in an effort to lose weight. This only results in poor diabetes control. Major adjustments to your insulin dose or diet are best made under professional guidance.

- Don't starve yourself or go on eating binges followed by purging. If you find yourself doing this, talk to a health professional about it immediately. Such behaviours can have devastating consequences for health.

- Don't be tempted to skip meals or snacks in an attempt to reduce your food intake. This not only upsets diabetes control and causes hypos but can leave you feeling very hungry and craving junk foods.

To lose weight eat well and be more active

Eat a well-balanced diet based on low G.I. food choices. Low G.I. foods have a beneficial effect on blood sugar control, are more sustaining and have a higher satiety value (that means they make you feel fuller for longer) compared with foods that have a high G.I. value.

Limit foods that are high in fat (such as chocolate, chips, biscuits, fried foods, potato crisps and cake).

Keep in contact with your health professional. As you lose weight, your insulin doses should be reviewed.

Do something active everyday. Increasing physical activity doesn't have to mean vigorous exercise. It simply means less time lying around.

Incorporate exercise into your daily routine. There are lots of options, from team sports to aerobics classes, swimming or gym. If you want something less structured, try walking, jogging, cycling or roller-blading. Studies have shown that people who achieve more than 12 500 'steps' per day don't gain weight over the long term, irrespective of what they eat. If you want to check out your own activity level, use a pedometer. It measures how many steps a day you achieve.

Being more active makes you look better
and feel better. Truly!

Juggling sporting commitments

Playing sport can provide enormous benefits to diabetes control and general wellbeing. To perform at your best, you need to monitor the effect playing sport has on your diabetes control, pay attention to diet and plan ahead. Remember to:

- ■ eat extra carbohydrate during periods of strenuous activity
- ■ exercise when levels of insulin are not peaking (although this is not always practical), and
- ■ inject insulin into an area that is not involved with the vigorous activity.

Coping with that early-morning training session before breakfast

Consume extra low G.I. carbohydrate before training – e.g. a bowl of Quick Oats. When you have finished training, take your insulin dose, then have your normal breakfast around the usual time.

Coping with training/competition during meal and snack times

Eat carbohydrate appropriate for the level of activity plus additional carbohydrate to allow for the delay in the mealtime. A combination of low and high G.I. foods would be best.

When you know you need additional carbohydrate before competing but have no appetite or desire to eat

Choose light foods or fluids that sit well in your stomach; for example, a banana smoothie, fruit salad or a banana.

Working part-time

If you have part-time work, you may need to alter your usual routine to fit in with your scheduled work breaks or negotiate adequate breaks with your employer.

Before starting work, have a substantial low G.I. meal or snack to help sustain your blood sugar levels. It may be a good idea to take extra carbohydrate snacks such as dried fruits, biscuits, muesli bars and fruit drinks from home so that you can eat them on the run. Sometimes small frequent snacks need to take the place of a full meal break. If the job is quite busy, make sure you are prepared with extra high G.I. carbohydrate snacks, or consider reducing your insulin dose.

DEAR HEATHER

I eat too much after school, then have high blood sugar readings and am never hungry at the evening meal.
You are hungry and eating large quantities for afternoon tea but the effects of your long-acting insulin are wearing off, hence the high blood sugar reading.

First, watch the foods you are eating for the afternoon snack. High fat snack foods, such as chips or biscuits, do not readily satisfy the appetite. Try combining them with some low G.I. foods that will satisfy your appetite and have a minimal impact on your blood sugar; for example, milk *and* a biscuit.

Try to work out why you are so hungry. Are you eating enough during the day? Providing low G.I. food choices throughout the day may help to alleviate your ravenous appetite after school.

Are you eating because you are bored? Once you've had your snack try to get out of the kitchen.

Alternatively, adjust your insulin regimen. Divide the pre-dinner insulin dose into two separate injections by giving the short-acting insulin after school. That way you'll have adequate insulin to cope with your large after-school appetite. The long-acting insulin may then be given before supper.

I am very active and attend football training three afternoons per week. I always eat extra foods before training but seem to hypo late evening after each session. Is there something more I should be doing?

Delayed hypoglycaemia after strenuous activity is usually an indication that either more carbohydrate or less insulin is required. Glucose stored in the liver may have been used during the activity and it is not until later in the evening, when the body tries to replenish its stores, that the hypo occurs. This can be prevented by taking more high G.I. carbohydrate prior to, during or immediately after the event. Alternatively, reduce your insulin dose if further increases in carbohydrate intake are not desired. Ensure that your evening meal and supper contain additional carbohydrate foods and are based on low G.I. food choices to sustain blood sugar levels overnight.

Appetite is often a good guide when determining additional carbohydrate needs. Eating extra low G.I. foods at dinner and/or supper to match the appetite after strenuous activities is recommended. Temporarily performing more frequent blood tests prior to, during, immediately after and 4–6 hours after the training sessions will give you more information on which to base decisions.

RECOMMENDED DAILY QUANTITIES OF FOOD FOR TEENAGERS

Food group	Suggested daily quantity
Bread and cereals (particularly wholegrain breads, low G.I. cereals, pasta, low G.I. rice)	4 or more servings
Fruit and vegetables (particularly low G.I. varieties)	5 or more servings
Meat and meat alternatives (particularly low G.I. legumes and pulses)	1–2 servings (200 g)
Milk and dairy foods	3 servings (600 ml)
Margarine and oils	1 tablespoon (20 g)

Try to include a minimum of one low G.I. food per meal per day to achieve good long-term diabetes control.

LOW G.I. SNACKS

For toddlers

Apricot muffin • Cup of milk and an oatmeal biscuit •
Frozen yoghurt • Fruit yoghurt • Raisin toast spread
lightly with low fat cream cheese • Slice of fresh low G.I.
bread with margarine and Marmite™ • Sliced apple •
Small bowl of dried fruit – apricot halves, dried apples
and sultanas

For school children

Canned fruit snack pack • Carrot, celery and zucchini
sticks with houmous dip • Cheese melted on low G.I.
toast • Frozen yoghurt on a stick • Fruit bun • Fruit plate
of sliced apple, orange rings, grapes or melon chunks •
Ice-cream in a cone • Mandarin or a bunch of grapes •
Mini corn cob • Quick cooking noodles • Savoury
muffin (try peppers, sweet corn and cheese) • Vegetable
soup with a crusty wholegrain roll • Yoghurt with fruit
and nuts

For teenagers

Apple or banana • Baked beans on toast • Crumpets,
muffins or raisin bread • Instant noodles • Leftovers –
pizza, rice, noodles • Low fat ice-cream and low fat milk
• Nachos – corn chips and melted cheese • Nutri-Grain™

• Pasta snack • Popcorn • Smoothie • Toasted sandwich with low G.I. bread

Sandwich suggestions
Tuna, creamed corn and lettuce • Egg, mayonnaise, celery and lettuce • Tuna, salmon or sardines • Cheese with Marmite™ or tomato • Cheese and salad with mayonnaise • Egg mayonnaise or curry • Pâté, or meat or fish pastes • Tahini or houmous • Peanut butter and honey • Cold meat with pickles and/or salad/coleslaw and mayonnaise • Baked beans, bean salad or spaghetti • Mashed banana • Grilled sausages or cooked frankfurters (hot dogs) • Avocado and fresh chicken • Cream cheese with dried fruits • Crispy bacon, avocado, tomato and lettuce • Grated apple and sultanas • Grated carrot and apple with cream cheese • Ham, pineapple and cheese muffin • Banana nutty roll (banana, peanut butter, yoghurt)

THE G.I. FACTOR MENU PLANNER
Breakfast

For toddlers

Porridge with sultanas and milk and a small glass of
orange juice

A fruit smoothie – strawberries or banana with milk,
yoghurt and honey

A small yoghurt with chopped fresh fruit

Scrambled eggs on toast with a small cup of juice or milk

Mini-Wheats with milk and sliced banana

Fruit toast with cinnamon and a cup of milk

Baked beans on toast with a small juice or milk

For school children

French toast, made by lightly soaking thick slices of bread
in beaten egg and milk and pan-frying in a little
vegetable oil. Sprinkle with cinnamon sugar.

A bowl of Mini-Wheats with sliced canned peaches and
low fat milk

Sliced banana topped with vanilla yoghurt and a sprinkle
of muesli

Marmite™ on low G.I. toast

Boiled egg, low G.I. toast and a glass of orange juice

English muffin topped with creamed corn and grated
cheese under the grill

For teenagers

Bagels

Banana on toast

Breakfast cereal with milk and fruit

Creamed corn on toast with cheese and pepper

French toast with fresh fruit

Fruit smoothie

Grilled tomato and cheese on toast/muffins

Muffin or crumpet with jam

Poached eggs on toast

Porridge and sultanas

Toasted wholegrain sandwich

Wholegrain toast with peanut butter, cheese, egg or
  baked beans

Yoghurt and fresh fruit

Lunch Boxes

Some tasty combinations

Pitta bread filled with grated cheese and tabbouleh
A fruit muffin
Small apple and orange juice

Chicken drumstick with cucumber sticks, cherry toma-
  toes and cracker biscuits
Frozen tub of flavoured yoghurt
Fruit and jelly snack pack

Rice salad with canned tuna, corn kernels and diced red
  peppers
Small container of fresh pineapple chunks
Frozen flavoured milk drink

Pitta bread spread with margarine and Marmite™, folded
  around a cheese slice
A fruit yoghurt
Small container of dried apricots, sultanas and peanuts

Half a pitta bread slice rolled around houmous, grated
  carrot, cheese and lettuce
Frozen fruit juice
Container of diced melon

Main Meals

Favourites with toddlers

Grilled cheese on wholegrain toast fingers and a sliced apple

Macaroni cheese

Sweet corn fritters

Tomato soup and low G.I. toast

Tuna chow mein – canned tuna with fine noodles, stir-fried cabbage, onion, shredded carrot and courgettes, seasoned with soy sauce

Vegetable soup with noodles

Other meal ideas

Vegetable parcels: combined chopped cooked broccoli, grated carrot, chopped shallots and sweet corn with ricotta cheese and grated cheddar. Wrap in filo pastry and bake until golden.

Bottled pasta sauce on pasta with a sprinkle of parmesan cheese

Casserole with chunky vegetables and sweet potato cubes served with Basmati rice or noodles

Fish kebabs: cubes of firm white fish fillets threaded with banana, pineapple and button mushrooms

Jacket potato topped with baked beans and grated mozzarella

Lentil and vegetable burger

Nachos or tacos with beef and bean topping, avocado, shredded lettuce, tomato and reduced fat grated cheddar

Stir-fried beef, chicken or fish served with Basmati rice or noodles

FOR PARENTS

■ When putting together school lunches, use different types of bread for variety: wholegrain, wholemeal, white, sourdough, rye, raisin, fruit loaf, muffins, pitta, cheese rolls, herb bread, cheese and bacon rolls, etc.

■ Whichever meal you're planning, try to select a low G.I. variety where practical to help lower the G.I. for the day.

■ Toasted sandwiches can be cooked the night before and eaten cool for lunch the next day to add interest to the lunch box.

JUST DESSERTS

Desserts are delicious and there's no need to do without them; in fact, they can make a valuable contribution to your daily calcium and vitamin C intake when they are based on low fat dairy foods and fruit. Here are some quick and easy low G.I. dessert ideas.

Apple pie or fruit strudel
Banana and chocolate custard
Canned fruit (peaches, pears or apricots) with ice-cream
    or custard
Creamed rice pudding
Frozen yoghurt
Fruit crumble
Fruit salad and yoghurt
Ice-cream and sprinkles
Jellied fruit and ice-cream
Jelly whip made with low fat milk or yoghurt and set with
    fruit
Low fat ice-cream and strawberries
Stewed fruit and yoghurt

HOW WE MEASURE THE G.I. FACTOR

Pure glucose produces the greatest rise in blood sugar levels. All other foods have less effect when fed in equal carbohydrate quantities. The G.I. of pure glucose is set at 100 and other foods are ranked on a scale from 0 to 100 according to their effect on blood sugar levels.

To find out the G.I. of a food, a volunteer eats an amount of that test food containing 50 grams of carbohydrate (calculated from food composition tables or measured in the laboratory) – 50 grams of carbohydrate is equivalent to 3 tablespoons of pure glucose powder.

Over the next 2 hours (3 hours if the volunteer has diabetes), we take a blood sample every 15 minutes during the first hour and every 30 minutes thereafter. We measure and record the blood sugar level of these samples.

The blood sugar level is plotted on a graph and the area under the curve is calculated using a computer program (see diagram).

We compare the volunteer's response to the test food with his/her blood sugar response to 50 grams of pure glucose (the reference food).

The reference food is tested on two or three separate occasions and we calculate an average value to reduce the effect of day-to-day variation in blood sugar responses.

Note: The G.I. factor of the test food is the average value of a group of eight to 12 volunteers. Results obtained in a group of people with diabetes are comparable to those without diabetes. We refer to all foods according to a standard where glucose equals 100.

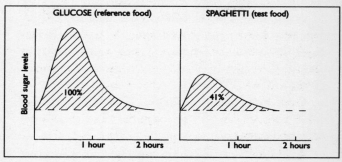

The effect of a food on blood sugar levels is calculated using the area under the curve (hatched area). The area under the curve after consumption of the test food is compared with the same area after the reference food (usually 50 grams of pure glucose).

HOW TO USE THE G.I. TABLES

These simplified tables are an A–Z listing of the G.I. factor of foods commonly eaten in Britain and Ireland. Approximately 300 different foods are listed.

The G.I. value shown next to each food is the average for that food using glucose as the standard; that is, glucose has a G.I. value of 100, with other foods rated accordingly. The average may represent the mean of 10 studies of that food worldwide or only two to four studies. In a few instances, British data are different to the rest of the world.

We have included some foods in the list which are not commonly eaten and other foods which may be encountered on overseas trips.

To check on a food's G.I., simply look for it by name in the alphabetic list. You may also find it under a food type – fruit, biscuits.

Included in the tables are the carbohydrate (CHO) and fat content of a sample serving of the food. This is to help you keep track of the amount of fat and carbohydrate in your diet. Refer to pages 12 and 14 for advice on how much carbohydrate and fat is recommended.

Remember, when choosing foods, that the G.I. factor isn't the only thing to consider. In terms of your blood sugar level you should also consider the amount of carbohydrate you are eating. For your overall health the fat, fibre and micronutrient content of your diet is also important. A dietitian can guide you further with good food choices.

Check our website for revised and new G.I. values: www.glycemicindex.com

A–Z OF FOODS
WITH G.I. FACTOR, PLUS
CARBOHYDRATE & FAT COUNTER

Food	G.I.	Fat	CHO
		(grams per serving)	
All Bran™, 40 g	42	1	22
Angel food cake, 30 g	67	trace	17
Apple, 1 medium, 150 g	38	0	18
Apple juice, unsweetened, 250 ml	40	0	33
Apple muffin, 1, 180 g	44	10	44
Apricots, fresh, 3 medium, 100 g	57	0	7
canned, light syrup, 125 g	64	0	13
dried, 5–6 pieces, 30 g	31	0	13
Bagel, 1 white, 70g	72	1	35
Baked beans, canned in tomato sauce, 120 g	48	1	13
Banana cake, 1 slice, 80 g	47	7	46
Banana, raw, 1 medium, 150 g	55	0	32
Barley, pearled, boiled, 80 g	25	1	17
Basmati white rice, boiled, 180 g	58	0	50
Beetroot, canned, drained, 2–3 slices, 60 g	64	0	5
Bengal gram dhal, 100g	54	5	57
Biscuits			
Digestives, plain, 2 biscuits, 30 g	59	6	21
Milk Arrowroot, 2 biscuits, 16 g	63	2	13

Food	G.I.	Fat	CHO
			(grams per serving)

Biscuits (*continued*)

Morning Coffee, 3 biscuits, 18 g	79	2	14
Oatmeal, 3 biscuits, 30 g	54	6	19
Rich Tea, 2 biscuits, 20 g	55	3	16
Shortbread, 2 biscuits, 30 g	64	8	19
Vanilla wafers, 6 biscuits, 30 g	77	5	21
Wheatmeal, 2 biscuits, 16 g	62	2	12
see *also* Crackers			
Black bean soup, 220 ml	64	2	82
Black beans, boiled, 120 g	30	1	26
Black gram, soaked and boiled, 120 g	43	1	16
Blackbread, dark rye, 1 slice, 50	76	1	21
Blackeyed beans, soaked, boiled, 120 g	42	1	24
Blueberry muffin, 1, 80 g	59	8	41
Bran			
Oat bran, 1 tablespoon, 10 g	55	1	7
Rice bran, extruded, 1 tablespoon, 10 g	19	2	3
Bran Buds™, breakfast cereal, 30 g	58	1	14
Bran muffin, 1, 80 g	60	8	34
Breads			
Dark rye, Blackbread, 1 slice, 50 g	76	1	21
Dark rye, Schinkenbröt, 1 slice, 50 g	86	1	22

Food	G.I.	Fat	CHO
		(grams per serving)	
Breads (*continued*)			
French baguette, 30 g	95	1	15
Fruit loaf, heavy, 1 slice, 35 g	47	1	18
Gluten-free bread, 1 slice, 30 g	90	1	14
Hamburger bun, 1 prepacked bun, 50 g	61	3	24
Light rye, 1 slice, 50 g	68	1	23
Linseed rye, 1 slice, 50 g	55	5	21
Melba toast, 4 squares, 30 g	70	1	19
Pitta bread, 1 piece, 65 g	57	1	38
Pumpernickel, 2 slices	41	2	35
Rye bread, 1 slice, 50 g	65	1	23
Sourdough rye, 1 slice, 50 g	57	2	23
Vogel's™, Honey & Oat loaf, 1 slice, 40 g	55	3	17
White (wheat flour), 1 slice, 30 g	70	1	15
Wholemeal (wheat flour), 1 slice, 35 g	69	1	14
Bread stuffing, 60 g	74	5	17
Breadfruit, 120 g	68	1	17
Breakfast cereals			
All-Bran™, 40 g	42	1	22
Bran Buds™, 30 g	58	1	14
Cheerios™, 30 g	74	2	20

Food	G.I.	Fat	CHO
		(grams per serving)	
Breakfast cereals (*continued*)			
Coco Pops™, 30 g	77	0	26
Cornflakes, 30 g	84	0	26
Mini Wheats™ (whole wheat), 30 g	58	0	21
Muesli, toasted, 60 g	43	9	33
Muesli, non-toasted, 60 g	56	6	32
Oat bran, raw, 1 tablespoon, 10 g	55	1	7
Porridge (cooked with water), 245 g	42	2	24
Puffed wheat, 30 g	80	1	22
Rice bran, 1 tablespoon, 10 g	19	2	3
Rice Krispies™, 30 g	82	0	27
Shredded wheat, 25 g	67	0	18
Special K™, 30 g	54	0	21
Sultana Bran™, 45 g	52	1	35
Sustain™, 30 g	68	1	25
Weetabix™, 2 biscuits, 30 g	69	1	19
Broad beans, frozen, boiled, 80 g	79	1	9
Buckwheat, cooked, 80 g	54	3	57
Bun, hamburger, 1 prepacked bun, 50 g	61	3	24
Burghel, cooked, 120 g	48	0	22
Butter beans, boiled, 70 g	31	0	13

Food	G.I.	Fat	CHO
		(grams per serving)	
Cakes			
Angel food cake, 1 slice, 30 g	67	trace	17
Banana cake, 1 slice, 80 g	47	7	46
Flan, 1 slice, 80 g	65	5	55
Pound cake, 1 slice, 80 g	54	15	42
Sponge cake, 1 slice, 60 g	46	16	32
Cantaloupe melon, raw, ¼ small, 200 g	65	0	6
Capellini pasta, boiled, 180 g	45	0	53
Carrots, peeled, boiled, 70 g	49	0	3
Cereal grains			
Barley, pearled, boiled, 80 g	25	1	17
Buckwheat, cooked, 80 g	54	3	57
Burghul, cooked, 120 g	48	0	22
Couscous, cooked, 120 g	65	0	28
Maize			
Cornmeal, wholegrain, cooked, 40 g	68	1	30
Sweet corn, canned, drained, 80 g	55	1	16
Taco shells, 2 shells, 26 g	68	6	16
Millet Ragi, cooked, 120 g	71	0	12
Rice			
Basmati, white, boiled, 180 g	58	0	50
Tapioca (boiled with milk), 250 g	81	10.5	51

Food	G.I.	Fat	CHO
		(grams per serving)	
Cheerios™, breakfast cereal, 30 g	74	2	20
Cherries, 20, 80 g	22	0	10
Chick peas, canned, drained, 95 g	42	2	15
Chick peas, boiled, 120 g	33	3	22
Chocolate, milk, 6 squares, 30 g	49	8	19
Coco Pops™, breakfast cereal, 30 g	77	0	26
Condensed milk, sweetened, ½ cup, 163 g	61	15	90
Corn bran, breakfast cereal, 30 g	75	1	20
Corn chips, Doritos™ original, 50 g	42	11	33
Cornflakes, breakfast cereal, 30 g	84	0	26
Cornmeal (maizemeal), cooked, 40 g	68	1	30
Couscous, cooked, 120 g	65	0	28
Crackers			
Premium soda crackers, 3 biscuits, 25 g	74	4	17
Puffed crispbread, 4 biscuits, wholemeal, 20 g	81	1	15
Rice cakes, 2 cakes, 25 g	82	1	21
Ryvita™, 2 slices, 20 g	69	1	16
Stoned wheat thins, 5 biscuits, 25 g	67	2	17
Water biscuits, 5, 25 g	78	2	18
Croissant, 1	67	14	27

Food	G.I.	Fat	CHO
		(grams per serving)	
Crumpet, 1, toasted, 50 g	69	0	22
Custard, 175 g	43	5	24
Dairy foods			
Ice cream, full fat, 2 scoops, 50 g	61	6	10
Ice cream, low fat, 2 scoops, 50 g	50	2	13
Milk, full fat, 250 ml	27	10	12
Milk, skimmed, 250 ml	32	0	13
Milk, chocolate flavoured, low-fat, 250 ml	34	3	23
Custard, 175 g	43	5	24
Yoghurt			
low-fat, fruit, 200 g	33	0	26
low-fat, artificial sweetener, 200 g	14	0	12
Dark rye bread, Blackbread, 1 slice, 50 g	76	1	21
Dark rye bread, Schinkenbröt, 1 slice, 50 g	86	1	22
Digestive biscuits, 2 plain, 30 g	59	6	21
Doughnut with cinnamon and sugar, 40 g	76	8	16
Fanta™, soft drink, 1 can, 375 ml	68	0	51
Fettucini, cooked, 180 g	32	1	57

Food	G.I.	Fat	CHO
			(grams per serving)
Fish fingers, oven-cooked, 5 × 25 g			
fingers, 125 g	38	14	24
Flan cake, 1 slice, 80 g	65	5	55
French baguette bread, 30 g	95	1	15
French fries, fine cut, small			
serving, 120 g	75	26	49
Fructose, pure, 10 g	23	0	10
Fruit cocktail, canned in natural			
juice, 125 g	55	0	15
Fruit loaf, heavy, 1 slice, 35 g	47	1	18
Fruits and fruit products			
Apple, 1 medium, 150 g	38	0	18
Apple juice, unsweetened, 250 ml	40	0	33
Apricots, fresh, 3 medium, 100 g	57	0	7
canned, light syrup, 125 g	64	0	13
dried, 5–6 pieces, 30 g	31	0	13
Banana, raw, 1 medium, 150 g	55	0	32
Cantaloupe melon, raw,			
¼ small, 200 g	65	0	10
Cherries, 20, 80 g	22	0	10
Fruit cocktail, canned in			
natural juice, 125 g	55	0	15
Grapefruit juice, unsweetened,			
250 ml	48	0	16
Grapefruit, raw, ½ medium, 100g	25	0	5

Food	G.I.	Fat	CHO
			(grams per serving)
Fruits and fruit products (*cont.*)			
Grapes, green, 100 g	46	0	15
Kiwifruit, 1 raw, peeled, 80 g	52	0	8
Lychee, canned and drained, 7, 90 g	79	0	16
Mango, 1 small, 150 g	55	0	19
Orange, 1 medium, 130 g	44	0	10
Orange juice, 250 ml	46	0	21
Pawpaw, ½ small, 200 g	58	0	14
Peach, fresh, 1 large, 110 g	42	0	7
canned, natural juice, 125 g	30	0	12
canned, heavy syrup, 125 g	58	0	19
canned, light syrup, 125 g	52	0	18
Pear, fresh, 1 medium, 150 g	38	0	21
canned in pear juice, 125 g	44	0	13
Pineapple, fresh, 2 slices, 125 g	66	0	10
Pineapple juice, unsweetened, canned, 250 ml	46	0	27
Plums, 3–4 small, 100 g	39	0	7
Raisins, 40 g	64	0	28

Food	G.I.	Fat	CHO
		(grams per serving)	
Fruits and fruit products (*cont.*)			
Sultanas, 40 g	56	0	30
Watermelon, 150 g	72	0	8
Gluten-free bread, 1 slice, 30 g	90	1	14
Glutinous rice, white, steamed, 1 cup, 174 g	98	0	37
Gnocchi, cooked, 145 g	68	0	71
Grapefruit juice, unsweetened, 250 ml	48	0	16
Grapefruit, raw, ½ medium, 100 g	25	0	5
Grape Nuts™ cereal, ½ cup, 58 g	71	1	47
Grapes, green, 100 g	46	0	15
Green gram dhal, 100 g	62	4	10
Green gram, soaked and boiled, 120 g	38	1	18
Green pea soup, canned, ready to serve, 220 ml	66	1	22
Hamburger bun, 1 prepacked, 50 g	61	3	24
Haricot (navy beans), boiled, 90 g	38	0	11
Honey & Oat Bread (Vogel's™), 1 slice, 40 g	55	3	17
Honey, 1 tablespoon, 20 g	58	0	16
Ice cream, full fat, 2 scoops, 50 g	61	6	10
Ice cream, low-fat, 2 scoops, 50 g	50	2	13
Jelly beans, 5, 10 g	80	0	9

Food	G.I.	Fat	CHO
			(grams per serving)
Kidney beans, boiled, 90 g	27	0	18
Kidney beans, canned and drained, 95 g	52	0	13
Kiwifruit, 1 raw, peeled, 80 g	52	0	8
Lactose, pure, 10 g	46	0	10
Lentil soup, canned, 220ml	44	0	14
Lentils, green and brown, dried, boiled, 95 g	30	0	16
Lentils, red, boiled, 120 g	26	1	21
Light rye bread, 1 slice, 50 g	68	1	23
Linguine pasta, thick, cooked, 180 g	46	1	56
Linguine pasta, thin, cooked, 180 g	55	1	56
Linseed rye bread, 1 slice, 50 g	55	5	21
Lucozade™, original, 1 bottle, 300 ml	95	<1	56
Lungkow bean thread, 180 g	26	0	61
Lychee, canned and drained, 7, 90 g	79	0	16
Macaroni cheese, packaged, cooked, 220 g	64	24	30
Macaroni, cooked, 180 g	45	1	56
Maize			
Cornmeal, wholegrain, 40 g	68	1	30
Sweet corn, canned and drained, 80 g	55	1	16

Food	G.I.	Fat	CHO
		(grams per serving)	
Maltose (maltodextrins), pure, 10 g	105	0	10
Mango, 1 small, 150 g	55	0	19
Mars Bar™, 60 g	68	11	41
Melba toast, 4 squares, 30 g	70	1	19
Milk, full fat, 250 ml	27	10	12
Milk, skimmed, 250 ml	32	0	13
chocolate flavoured, 250 ml	34	3	23
Milk, sweetened condensed,			
½ cup, 160 g	61	15	90
Milk Arrowroot biscuits, 2, 16 g	63	2	13
Millet, cooked, 120 g	71	0	12
Mini Wheats™ (whole wheat)			
breakfast cereal, 30 g	58	0	21
Morning Coffee biscuits, 3, 18 g	79	2	14
Muesli bars with fruit, 30 g	61	4	17
Muesli, breakfast cereal			
toasted, 60 g	43	9	33
non-toasted, 60 g	56	6	32
Muffins			
Apple, 1 muffin, 80 g	44	10	44
Bran, 1 muffin, 80 g	60	8	34
Blueberry, 1 muffin, 80 g	59	8	41
Mung bean noodles, 1 cup, 140 g	39	0	35
Noodles, 2-minute, 85 g packet,			
cooked	46	16	55

Food	G.I.	Fat	CHO
			(grams per serving)
Noodles, rice, fresh, boiled, 1 cup 176 g	40	0	44
Oat bran, raw, 1 tablespoon, 10 g	55	1	7
Oatmeal biscuits, 3 biscuits, 30 g	54	6	19
Orange, 1 medium, 130 g	44	0	10
Orange juice, 250 ml	46	0	21
Orange squash, diluted, 250 ml	66	0	20
Parsnips, boiled, 75 g	97	0	8
Pasta			
Capellini, cooked, 180 g	45	0	53
Fettucini, cooked, 180 g	32	1	57
Gnocchi, cooked, 145 g	68	3	71
Noodles, 2-minute, 85 g packet, cooked	46	16	55
Linguine, thick, cooked, 180 g	46	1	56
Linguine, thin, cooked, 180 g	55	1	56
Macaroni cheese, packaged, cooked, 200g	64	24	30
Macaroni, cooked, 180 g	45	1	56
Noodles, mung bean, 1 cup, 140 g	39	0	35
Noodles, rice, fresh, boiled, 1 cup, 176 g	40	0	44
Ravioli, meat-filled, cooked, 220g	39	11	30

Food	G.I.	Fat	CHO
			(grams per serving)
Pasta (*continued*)			
Rice pasta, brown, cooked, 180 g	92	2	57
Spaghetti, white, cooked, 180 g	41	1	56
Spaghetti, wholemeal, cooked, 180 g	37	1	48
Spirale, durum, cooked, 180 g	43	1	56
Star pastina, cooked, 180 g	38	1	56
Tortellini, cheese, cooked, 180 g	50	8	21
Vermicelli, cooked, 180 g	35	0	45
Pastry, flaky, 65 g	59	26	25
Pawpaw, raw, ½ small, 200 g	58	0	14
Pea and ham soup, canned, 220 ml	66	2	13
Peach, fresh, 1 large, 110 g	42	0	7
canned, natural juice, 125 g	30	0	12
canned, heavy syrup, 125 g	58	0	19
canned, light syrup, 125 g	52	0	18
Peanuts, roasted, salted, 75 g	14	40	11
Pear, fresh, 1 medium, 150 g	38	0	21
canned in pear juice, 125 g	44	0	13
Peas, green, fresh, frozen, boiled 80 g	48	0	5
Peas, dried, boiled, 70 g	22	0	4

Food	G.I.	Fat	CHO
		(grams per serving)	
Pineapple, fresh, 2 slices, 125 g	66	0	10
Pineapple juice, unsweetened, canned, 250 g	46	0	27
Pinto beans, canned, 95 g	45	0	13
Pinto beans, soaked, boiled, 90 g	39	0	20
Pitta bread, 1 piece, 65 g	57	1	38
Pizza, cheese and tomato, 2 slices, 230 g	60	27	57
Plums, 3–4 small, 100 g	39	0	7
Popcorn, low-fat (popped), 20 g	55	2	10
Porridge (made with water), 245 g	42	2	24
Potatoes			
French fries, fine cut, small serving, 120 g	75	26	49
instant potato	83	1	18
new, peeled, boiled, 5 small (cocktail), 175 g	62	0	23
new, canned, drained, 5 small 175 g	61	0	20
pale skin, peeled, boiled, 1 medium, 120 g	56	0	16
pale skin, baked in oven (no fat), 1 medium, 120 g	85	0	14
pale skin, mashed, 120 g	70	0	16

Food	G.I.	Fat	CHO
			(grams per serving)
Potatoes (*continued*)			
pale skin, steamed, 1 medium, 120 g	65	0	17
pale skin, microwaved, 1 medium, 120 g	82	0	17
potato crisps, plain, 50 g	54	16	24
Potato crisps, plain, 50 g	54	16	24
Pound cake, 1 slice, 80 g	54	15	42
Pretzels, 50 g	83	1	22
Puffed crispbread, 4 wholemeal, 20 g	81	1	15
Puffed wheat breakfast cereal, 30 g	80	1	22
Pumpernickel bread, 2 slices	41	2	35
Pumpkin, peeled, boiled, 85 g	75	0	6
Raisins, 40 g	64	0	28
Ravioli, meat-filled, cooked, 20 g	39	11	30
Rice			
Basmati, white, boiled, 180 g	58	0	50
Glutinous, white, steamed, 1 cup, 174 g	98	0	37
Instant, cooked, 180 g	87	0	38
Rice bran, extruded, 1 tablespoon, 10 g	19	2	3
Rice cakes, 2, 25 g	82	1	21
Rice Krispies™, breakfast cereal, 30 g	82	0	27

Food	G.I.	Fat	CHO
		(grams per serving)	
Rice noodles, fresh boiled, 1 cup, 176 g	40	0	44
Rice pasta, brown, cooked, 180 g	92	2	57
Rice vermicelli, cooked, 180 g	58	0	58
Rich Tea biscuits, 2, 20	55	3	16
Rye bread, 1 slice, 50 g	65	1	23
Ryvita™ crackers, 2 biscuits, 20 g	69	1	16
Sausages, fried, 2, 120 g	28	21	6
Semolina, cooked, 230 g	55	0	17
Shortbread, 2 biscuits, 30 g	64	8	19
Shredded wheat breakfast cereal, 25 g	67	0	18
Soda crackers, 3 biscuits, 25 g	74	4	17
Soft drink, Coca Cola™, 1 can, 375 ml	63	0	40
Soft drink, Fanta™, 1 can, 375 ml	68	0	51
Soups			
Black bean soup, 220 ml	64	2	82
Green pea soup, canned, ready to serve, 220 ml	66	1	22
Lentil soup, canned, 220 ml	44	0	14
Pea and ham soup, 220 ml	60	2	13
Tomato soup, canned, 220 ml	38	1	15
Sourdough rye bread, 1 slice, 50 g	57	2	23
Soya beans, canned, 100 g	14	6	12

Food	G.I.	Fat	CHO (grams per serving)
Soya beans, boiled, 90 g	18	7	10
Spaghetti, white, cooked, 180 g	41	1	56
Spaghetti, wholemeal, cooked 180 g	37	1	48
Special K™, 30 g	54	0	21
Spirale pasta, durum, cooked, 180 g	43	1	56
Split pea soup, 220 ml	60	0	6
Split peas, yellow, boiled, 90 g	32	0	16
Sponge cake plain, 1 slice, 60 g	46	16	32
Sports drinks			
Gatorade, 250 ml	78	0	15
Isostar, 250 ml	70	0	18
Stoned wheat thins, crackers, 5 biscuits, 25 g	67	2	17
Sucrose, 1 teaspoon	65	0	5
Sultana Bran™, 45 g	52	1	35
Sultanas, 40 g	56	0	30
Sustain™, 30 g	68	1	25
Swede, peeled, boiled, 60 g	72	0	3
Sweet corn, 85 g	55	1	16
Sweet potato, peeled, boiled, 80 g	54	0	16
Sweetened condensed milk, ½ cup, 160 g	61	15	90
Taco shells, 2, 26 g	68	6	16

Food	G.I.	Fat	CHO
		(grams per serving)	
Tapioca pudding, boiled with milk, 250 g	81	10.5	51
Tapioca, steamed 1 hour, 100 g	70	6	54
Tofu frozen dessert (non-dairy), 100 g	115	1	13
Tomato soup, canned, 220 ml	38	1	15
Tortellini, cheese, cooked, 180 g	50	8	21
Vanilla wafer biscuits, 6, 30 g	77	5	21
Vermicelli, cooked, 180 g	35	0	45
Waffles, 25 g	76	3	9
Water biscuits, 5, 25 g	78	2	18
Watermelon, 150 g	72	0	8
Weetabix™ breakfast cereal,2 biscuits, 30 g	69	1	19
Wheatmeal biscuits, 2, 16 g	62	2	12
White bread, wheat flour, 1 slice, 30 g	70	1	15
Wholemeal bread, wheat flour, 1 slice, 35 g	69	1	14
Yakult, 65 ml serving	46	0	11
Yam, boiled, 80 g	51	0	26
Yoghurt			
low-fat, fruit, 200 g	33	0	26
low-fat, artificial sweetener, 200 g	14	0	12

WHERE TO GO FOR HELP AND FURTHER INFORMATION

British Dietetic Association
5th Floor, Elizabeth House
22 Suffolk Street
Queensway
Birmingham B1 1LS
Telephone: (0121) 616 4900

British Diabetic Association
10 Queen Anne Street
London W1M 0BD
Telephone: (020) 7323 1531

Irish Nutrition & Dietetic Institute
Dundrum Business Centre
Frankfort Dundrum
Dublin 14
Ireland
Telephone: (+353 1) 298 7466

ABOUT THE AUTHORS

Associate Professor Jennie Brand-Miller, a member of the teaching and research staff of the Human Nutrition Unit at the University of Sydney, is a world authority on the glycaemic index of foods and its applications to diabetes.

Kaye Foster-Powell, an accredited practising dietitian-nutritionist, has extensive experience in diabetes management and has researched practical applications of the glycaemic index. She is the senior dietitian at Wentworth Area Diabetes Service and conducts a private practice in the Blue Mountains, New South Wales.

Heather Gilbertson, an accredited practising dietitian and diabetes educator, has extensive experience in diabetes management in children and adolescents and has researched the effect of low G.I. and measured carbohydrate diets in children with diabetes. She currently works at the Royal Children's Hospital Women's and Children's Health Care Network, Melbourne and conducts a private practice in the Macedon Ranges, Victoria.

Dr Anthony Leeds is Senior Lecturer in the Department of Nutrition and Dietetics at King's College London. He graduated in medicine from the Middlesex Hospital Medical School, London, UK in 1971. He conducts research on carbohydrate and dietary fibre in relation to heart disease, obesity and diabetes and continues part-time medical practice. He chairs the research ethics committee of King's College London, is a member of the Society of Authors, and in 1999 was elected a Fellow of the Institute of Biology.